WHAT THE FLUSH?!

NO YOU ARE NOT CRAZY IT'S JUST PERIMENOPAUSE

DR. AMU SUB

First Edition, 2025
Imprint: Independently published

For every woman who has ever wondered,
"Is it just me?"
No, it's not.
You are not broken.
You are powerful, worthy, and evolving — even in the chaos.

To my daughter —
May you walk into womanhood armed with knowledge, not shame.

To my mother —
You did the best you could with what you had. I see you now.

Table of Contents

Part 1: Breaking the Silence — Understanding Perimenopause

Chapter 1: The Ceremony, the Silence and the Shift

- Cultural taboos and myths
- Why We Don't Talk About This Enough
- The emotional toll of feeling "invisible"
- From daughter to Mother
- Rewriting the Story

Chapter 2: What's Happening to My Body?

- Understanding Perimenopause
- Menstrual changes
- When it's just PMS... and when it's perimenopause

Chapter 3: The Surprise of Starting Early

- The transitional phase of perimenopause
- Why is it happening?
- The importance of recognizing it early

Part 2: Living Through It — Practical Strategies

Chapter 4: Managing the Rollercoaster of Emotions

- Anxiety, rage, sadness: The emotional spectrum

- Coping strategies (mindfulness, therapy, journaling, community support)

Chapter 5: Taking Control of Your Body

- Weight changes, bloating, and that stubborn belly fat
- Exercise routines that help
- Supplements, diet tweaks, and the science behind them

Chapter 6: Sex, Intimacy, and Libido — The Untold Struggles

- Open discussion about vaginal dryness, pain, and libido shifts
- The grief of a lost sex drive
- Medical treatments vs natural options
- Rekindling intimacy

Chapter 7: Lost in the Fog

- Why can't I remember things?
- The science behind brain fog
- The real-life impact

Chapter 8: Fatigue, Freezing and Falling Apart

- Common mimickers
- What does research say?
- Significance of the thyroid and iron in perimenopause

Chapter 9: The Gallbladder Surprise

- Gallstones
- Research insight
- Hidden link

Chapter 10: The symptoms No One Warns You About

- Real struggles
- Recurrent UTIs
- Allergies
- Joint pains
- Dizziness and Palpitations

Part 3: Treatment Choices — Navigating the Options

Chapter 11: Why managing Perimenopause Matters

- Hormone chaos
- Weigt gain and metabolic syndrome
- Sleep disorder and OSA
- Mood disorders in perimenopause
- Bone health and osteoporosis

Chapter 12: Alternative and Complementary Therapies

- Acupuncture, meditation, and yoga
- Busting myths about "miracle cures"

- This Isn't the End — It's a New Beginning
- A final empowering message about embracing midlife with grace and power

INTRODUCTION

A final empowering message about embracing midlife with grace and power

This Is Not the End — It's the Beginning.

Because fighting something without knowing what it is, isn't a fair battle.

And let's be honest — so much about our biology and genetics is outside our control. We didn't choose our hormone blueprint. We didn't choose our menstrual cycles, our ovaries, or the timeline of our fertility. But here's what we can choose:

How we eat.
How we sleep.
How we nurture ourselves..

Perimenopause is not "just a phase." And it is certainly not "just perimenopause."

It is a powerful, often chaotic transition. It reshapes how we think, feel, move, sleep, connect, and exist. For many of us, it sneaks in quietly — disguised as exhaustion, irritability, or forgetfulness — until suddenly, we don't feel like ourselves anymore.

Here's the truth: Perimenopause is not the enemy.
It's not something going wrong — it's something happening exactly as nature intended.

The only problem? It doesn't follow the timeline.
It doesn't follow the rules.
It arrives unannounced and often overstays its welcome.

We live in a world where women are expected to juggle everything and still smile. We carry the invisible load — physically, emotionally, mentally — and we make it look easy.

And that's the problem.

Because when we make it look easy, so no one offers help. And when we do ask for help, we feel like we're failing.

But let me clear, **asking for help is not weakness.**

You don't have to be Superwoman. You don't have to hold it all together. You don't need to wait until you're on the edge of burnout to claim rest, support, or answers.

You're allowed to slow down.
You're allowed to prioritise your wellbeing.
You're allowed to say, "I'm not okay," and know that it doesn't make you any less strong — it makes you real, it makes you human.

This book exists to give you something I wish I had: a guide.

A voice that says, "You're not crazy."

A map that explains what's happening to your body and your brain.

And above all, a reminder that this isn't the end of you — it's the beginning of a more powerful, self-aware, and intentional you.

You can't change your biology, but you can work with it.

You can learn what's happening inside your body and respond with compassion instead of frustration.

You can honour the shifts, adapt your habits, and build a life that supports who you're becoming — not just who you were.

Your cup needs to be full before you can fill everyone else's.

You deserve to feel whole.
You deserve clarity, strength, and support.

This is not the end.

This is the re-introduction to you.

Welcome to the beginning.

Chapter 1: The Ceremony, the Silence, and the Shift

Shame, Sarees, and the Surprise of Bleeding in a Patriarchal Parade

In many cultures, especially mine, being a woman comes with a long list of unspoken rules, bizarre rituals, and hush-hush expectations. I'm a third-generation Malaysian woman of Indian heritage. In our household, menstruation was something you didn't talk about — unless, of course, the entire neighbourhood needed to know about it.

Let me explain.

I was 11 years old. A tomboy with short hair, scraped knees, and an identity crisis revolving around trying to outdo my older brother in every way imaginable. I love my brother and wanted to be exactly like him. I had no idea what a uterus was doing in my body, and certainly no plans for it to start bleeding.

But one sunny afternoon, life decided to hand me the crimson envelope. I had no cramps, no warning signs — just "what the hell is this?" in my undies. I did what any confused kid would do. I panicked. Then I told my mother.

That was a mistake. Or was it? How would I know?

Welcome to the Menstrual Circus

The next thing I knew, my house transformed overnight from modest family home to Bollywood bridal set. Ok, this is a little exaggeration on my part. It was 2 weeks after the eventful day that relatives I'd never met appeared out of thin air. Aunties (the kind you only see at funerals or weddings) flocked to my house in a blur of silk sarees, heavy jewellery, and unsolicited life advice. There were flower garlands, trays of sweets more people that I half-expected a band and a buffet.

All this… because I got my period.

In South Indian Tamil tradition, this was my *Sadangu* — also known as *Ritu Kala Samskara*. It's a sacred "coming-of-age" ceremony to honour a girl's first period. In theory, it celebrates the start of fertility and the girl's readiness to take her place in the adult female world. It's meant to be a joyful and empowering transition.

In practice? It felt like a hormonal ambush.

They dressed me in a saree, or two, even though I had no idea how to walk in one without tripping over myself. I had fake hair braided into my short crop, drowned in jasmine flowers. My face was powdered, rouged, and blushed until I looked like an undercooked drag queen. And worst of all, there was a photographer, who was my brother, and every time I looked at him, he kept giving me the proudest smile, and I felt even more betrayed. Yes. There is proof of all of this. I think I destroyed them all.

The entire human race seemed packed into my house. Cameras flashed. Relatives clapped. And some whispered about how I'd now "entered womanhood." I didn't even know where the blood came from, and yet here I was being treated like I was ready to marry a prince and bear five children.

Isolation, Eggs, and Ovarian Preservation

There's another part of this ritual people don't talk about much: the **isolation**. Once I got my period, I wasn't allowed to see the male members of my family. Not even my own father. I had to eat separately. Sit separately. And in some households — thankfully not mine — girls weren't even allowed to touch anything in the kitchen.

I was also given a "special diet" — supposedly to strengthen my uterus and ovaries. This included swallowing **raw kampung (village) eggs with gingerly oil (sesame oil)**, every morning. I gagged. Every. Single. Time.

Then came the ritual baths. Several aunties took turns bathing me with turmeric water, whispering prayers and mantras to bless my transition. That part I didn't mind. It was soothing, sacred even. I didn't fully understand it, but I appreciated the care behind it.

This whole process, I later learned, is rooted in Ayurvedic and Siddha medical traditions — believed to protect a girl's reproductive health and cleanse her body. It was also a social announcement: "She is now fertile." A sentence no 11-year-old needs broadcasted like a Facebook status, and thank god there was no social media in the 90's.

Why Was *Sadangu* Practiced in South India?

Historically, *Sadangu* served several purposes:

- To celebrate and support the girl entering womanhood

- To educate her about menstrual hygiene and fertility (although let's be honest, no one explained anything to me)
- To mark her eligibility for marriage in traditional settings
- To give her a social rite of passage and a sense of identity

In ancient times, when education and healthcare were less accessible, rituals like these were seen as a way to honour and guide young girls into a new phase of life.

But today? **We've carried forward the ritual, but not the reason.**
We hold the celebration, but skip the conversation.

Why We Never Spoke About It Again

After that grand production, you'd think someone would check in with me. But nope. Not a word. My mother, bless her soul, just gave me a packet of pads and told me to change it every few hours and not to tell anyone if I leaked, (and that leak happened A LOT throughout the years. We didn't have extra-long pads with wings those days!! It was an absolute horror and super embarrassing). So that was it. That was the entire manual.

Years passed. I went through medical school, studied reproductive physiology, and began practising as a GP. I could now explain ovulation, oestrogen, and the endometrial lining in five languages and under anaesthesia.(I only speak 3). But strangely, even with all that knowledge, I never thought about perimenopause.

I assumed menopause was for "older women." Like my grandmother. It didn't cross my mind that the weird emotional tsunamis, brain fog, and ragey episodes I started having in my 30s had anything to do with my hormones.

Why would I? We never talked about this stuff. Not then. Not now.

Full Circle — From Daughter to Mother

Here's the part I want to share most: **I did the exact same ceremony for my daughter** when she got her first period.

Yes — the same *Sadangu* that once made me feel confused, embarrassed, and out of control. But this time, **I changed the script**.

I never isolated her.
I never told her she was "dirty."
I made sure her father and brother supported her the entire time — because menstruation is not something to hide from the men in the family. It's something they should understand too.

I explained everything to her, **before it happened** — what a period is, what changes to expect, and what it means for her body. I made sure she knew this wasn't a curse, (who am I kidding, of course it's a curse, but she doesn't have to know that, not now) but a normal healthy milestone in her life. And I stood by her side for every step of the journey.

Her ceremony? It was **grand**. But this time, the girl at the centre of it all was **smiling**. She was **prepared**. She was **in control**.

She chose her attire — something culturally appropriate, but entirely *her*. She picked the colour. She chose how she wanted her makeup done. And when she stood there, surrounded by family and love, she didn't look like a confused child being paraded for others.

She looked like a young woman who understood her body — and felt proud of it.

And me? I cried. Not from confusion or shame. But from a quiet, deep, soul-anchored pride.

Because I realised something that day: **my mother did what she could for me with what she had**. She didn't have the words. She didn't have the knowledge. But she had the love. She wanted to honour me in the best way she knew how.

And now, as a mother, I was doing the same — with more tools, more knowledge, and a vow to make sure my daughter felt seen, heard, and empowered.

Because this is how change happens.
Not by burning rituals to the ground.
But by lighting them up with **understanding, education, and compassion.**

Let's Rewrite the Story

That coming-of-age ceremony wasn't the problem. The silence was.

And now, as I sit here — writing this book, healing my
inner child, guiding my patients, and watching my daughter
grow — I know something for sure:

We don't need less culture.
We need more conversation.

We don't need to stop celebrating womanhood.
We just need to start explaining it.

So let's talk.

About periods.
About perimenopause.
About pelvic floors and dried-up vaginas and forgotten
keys and emotional breakdowns over burnt toast.

Let's laugh about it, cry about it, and finally — finally —
stop feeling alone in it.

Because it's not dirty.
It's not shameful.
It's not something to whisper about in corners.

It's our biology.
It's our strength.
It's our story.

And girl — **it's time we rewrote it.**

Chapter 2: What's Happening to My Body?

Understanding the Rollercoaster of Perimenopause

When I was younger, I thought womanhood was simple: you had your period, and one day, it stopped. That was menopause — the end of the story. No one warned me about the **confusing, unpredictable, and emotionally draining** chapter in between: **perimenopause**.

If you're in your late 30s or 40s and feel like you're unravelling for no reason — you're not losing your mind. You're likely in **perimenopause**. And you're not alone.

Perimenopause — The Change Before The Change

Perimenopause means "around menopause." It's the transitional phase when your ovaries start slowing down, and your hormone levels — particularly **oestrogen and progesterone** — start to **fluctuate wildly**. These changes can begin as early as your mid-30s and last up to 10 years before your periods officially stop.

Once you've gone 12 consecutive months without a period, you're in **menopause**. But perimenopause is the *storm* before the still — and it's where most of the chaos happens. Isn't that just great, and here I thought having my period for the first time was a shocker.

Why Is This Happening?

Think of your ovaries like a light bulb that's dimming —
not switching off suddenly. As your ovarian reserve
declines, your hormones begin misfiring in surges and
slumps. This hormonal turbulence affects more than just
your period:

- **Mood**
- **Sleep**
- **Energy**
- **Memory**
- **Skin, hair, and bones**
- Even your **bladder and digestion**

That's why symptoms can feel all over the place —
because your hormones regulate almost *everything.*

Common Symptoms of Perimenopause

Perimenopause doesn't look the same for everyone. Some
women have just a few subtle shifts. Others feel like a
stranger has taken over their body.

Here's what you might experience:
Physical Symptoms

- Irregular or heavier periods
- Hot flushes or night sweats
- Breast tenderness
- Weight gain (especially belly)
- Fatigue or low energy

Physical Symptoms

- Joint or muscle aches
- Acne or thinning hair
- Sleep disturbances

Emotional / Cognitive Symptoms

- Mood swings, irritability
- Anxiety or panic attacks
- Brain fog or forgetfulness
- Low motivation, detachment
- Depression or persistent sadness
- Loss of libido
- Overwhelm, poor concentration
- Difficulty finding words or focusing

You might have just a few of these — or a full cocktail.

What's Going on with My Period?

This is often one of the first signs. Here's what to watch for:

- Shorter or longer cycles (e.g. every 21 or 40 days instead of 28)
- Heavier bleeding or passing clots
- Spotting between periods
- Periods that come out of nowhere

Eventually, your periods become more sporadic before stopping altogether.

When Does It Start?

Most women begin perimenopause between **ages 40 and 45**, but it can start earlier — even as early as **35** — especially if you've had children later, have high stress levels, or a family history of early menopause.

You're not imagining it. And no, **you're not too young**.

What About Blood Tests?

Perimenopause is mostly diagnosed **based on symptoms**, not blood tests — because hormone levels fluctuate **day to day**. That said, bloods can help rule out other causes of fatigue or irregular periods.

Your doctor might order:

- **FSH and oestradiol** (if early menopause is suspected)
- **TSH** (thyroid issues can mimic perimenopause)
- **Iron, Vitamin B12, and Vitamin D** (to exclude deficiency)
- **FBC** (if heavy bleeding or fatigue is present)

Don't be surprised if your hormone levels are "normal" one day and menopausal the next — that's the **hormonal chaos** of this phase.

When It's Just PMS… and When It's More

PMS happens predictably, usually right before your period, and resolves shortly after.

Perimenopausal mood swings, however, are:

- More intense
- Less predictable
- Often unrelated to your cycle
- Accompanied by other physical symptoms like hot flushes or sleep issues

If you find yourself crying at TV commercials, rage-cleaning the kitchen, or struggling to remember your child's teacher's name — that's not just PMS. That's perimenopause knocking.

You're Not Broken

This stage can feel like a loss of identity. You might wonder where the confident, clear-headed version of you has gone. But please know this:

You are not broken.
You are not weak.
You are **transitioning.**

Just like puberty, this is another biological shift. But this time, you're entering it with the wisdom, resilience, and self-awareness that only lived experience can bring.

"You're not fading — you're transforming."

OVULATORY CYCLE

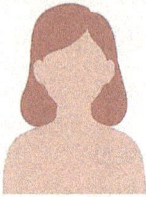

PUBERTY

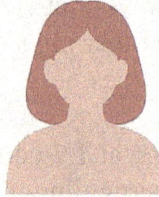

PERIMENOPAUSE

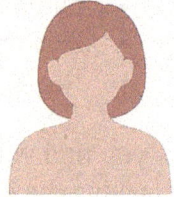

MENOPAUSE

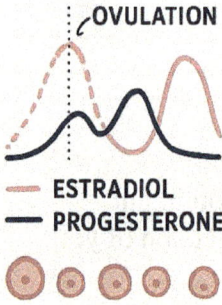

OVULATION

— ESTRADIOL
— PROGESTERONE

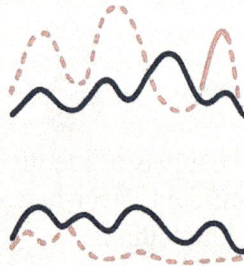

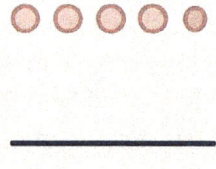

PUBERTY   **PERIMENOPAUSE**   **MENOPAUSE**

Chapter 3: The Surprise of Starting Early — When the Shift Comes Before You're Ready

I always thought menopause was something I'd worry about in my 50s. That's what the textbooks said. That's what my patients believed. That's what I believed — until it happened to me.

I was 35. A mother. A medical practitioner and a practice owner. A woman juggling her career, family, studies, and expectations. Life was busy, but manageable — or so I thought.

Then came the slow unravelling.

I started forgetting simple things. I couldn't find my words. I was always tired. My skin became dry, my cycles were painful, and I found myself in tears over things that never used to move me and I was angry over the smallest things. My usual ability to "push through" was no match for the storm that had arrived uninvited.

Looking back now, I realise: **this was perimenopause** — and I had no idea it started this early.

What Is Perimenopause?

Perimenopause is the **transitional phase before menopause**, when the body begins to shift from a reproductive to a non-reproductive state. It often begins in the **mid-to-late 30s or early 40s**, though many women — like myself — are caught off guard by how early and how intensely it begins.

It's not just a few skipped periods. It's not just some mood swings. It's a **complex neuroendocrine transformation** that can affect **every major system in your body**.

And no one talks about it enough.

Why Does Perimenopause Happen? — The Physiology

Here's what's going on under the surface:

Physiological Process	Impact
• Declining ovarian follicle reserve	Fewer follicles → irregular ovulation and menstrual cycles
• Fluctuating oestradiol levels	Sudden highs and lows → mood swings, hot flushes, anxiety
• Progesterone drops first	Unopposed oestrogen → heavy bleeding, irritability
• Neuroendocrine disruption	Brain-ovary signalling becomes erratic → hormonal chaos
• Other hormones impacted	Cortisol, insulin, thyroid may become dysregulated

This hormonal seesaw is why perimenopause feels like an identity crisis — physically, mentally, and emotionally.

Why Is It Happening Earlier Now?

You're not imagining it: **perimenopause is starting earlier** for many women.

Contributing factors include:

- **Chronic stress** → impacts the hypothalamic-pituitary-ovarian (HPO) axis
- **Environmental toxins** → endocrine-disrupting chemicals in plastics and cosmetics
- **Sleep disruption** → poor circadian rhythms from shift work or screen exposure
- **Nutrient depletion** → crash dieting and overtraining
- **Smoking and alcohol** → accelerates ovarian ageing
- **Earlier menarche** → more total ovulations = faster ovarian reserve depletion

Note: Earlier perimenopause doesn't necessarily mean earlier menopause — but it *does* mean you may spend more years navigating the symptoms if left untreated.

What Does the Research Say?

- **SWAN Study (US)**: Cognitive, mood, and physical symptoms peak during perimenopause. Chronic stress exacerbates them.

- **Epperson et al., 2013 (JAMA Psychiatry)**: Linked perimenopause with brain function changes, including reduced verbal memory.
- **Harvard Nurses' Health Study**: Healthy lifestyle choices can delay menopause and ease symptom severity.
- **AMS & NAMS Guidelines**: Perimenopause is a critical "**clinical window of opportunity**" to prevent long-term risks like osteoporosis, cardiovascular disease, and major depression.

Why It's So Important to Recognise Perimenopause Early

So many women are:

- Misdiagnosed with depression instead of hormone-driven mood changes
- Treated for abnormal uterine bleeding without understanding the hormonal cause
- Gaslit or dismissed when they say "something doesn't feel right"

Recognising **perimenopause for what it is** can lead to:

- Early and personalised intervention (HRT or non-hormonal treatments)
- Reduced risk of long-term chronic disease
- Empowered self-advocacy and mental clarity

How "Early Onset" Symptoms Differ from Textbook Menopause

Textbooks say menopause is hot flushes, night sweats, and no more periods. But **early perimenopause** isn't that clean-cut. It's subtler — and therefore easier to overlook:

Textbook Menopause
- No periods for 12 months
- Classic hot flushes
- Loss of libido
- Clear menopausal blood tests

Real-World Early Perimenopause
- Periods become shorter, heavier, unpredictable
- Silent anxiety, rage, internal heat, insomnia
- Emotional detachment, brain fog, crying without cause
- Normal hormones… but abnormal symptoms

In Summary: Perimenopause Isn't a Pause — It's a Shift

Aspect	Explanation
When it starts	Often between ages 35–45, sometimes even earlier
What's happening	Hormonal instability, brain-body miscommunication

Aspect	Explanation
Symptoms	Irregular cycles, mood swings, fatigue, brain fog, insomnia
Long-term risks	Osteoporosis, cardiovascular disease, diabetes, severe depression
Why earlier now?	Stress, environmental exposures, poor sleep, early menarche
What helps?	Early diagnosis, lifestyle changes, HRT if appropriate

"This isn't you losing control. It's your body transitioning. You're not fading — you're transforming."

Chapter 4: Managing the Rollercoaster of Emotions

From Rage to Relief — Finding Calm in the Chaos

Between the ages of 35 to 40, I didn't suspect perimenopause — not even a little. What I did know was that **emotionally, I was unravelling**.

The rage. The sadness. The tears that came out of nowhere. It wasn't just mood swings — it was like an emotional hijacking. And the worst part? It often landed right on the person I loved the most: my husband.

Every little thing he did — or didn't do — would set me off. I wasn't someone who yelled or lost control. But suddenly, I was shouting, crying, or retreating into a shell I didn't recognise. I felt ashamed, exhausted, and confused. Who *was* this person?

Then COVID hit.

With clinics slowing down and the world on pause, I had time — too much time. That stillness made me realise: **something needed to change, and it had to start with me.** You won't believe it, while I was home bound with my 2 children, my husband was locked in a room due to COVID quarantine, I picked up crocheting. I made a unicorn out of yarn and somehow, in that quiet repetitive motion, I began to find **myself again**. I also learned to meditate and that was how my life changed.

"An idle mind is the devil's playground. A calm, busy one is your anchor in the storm."

The Emotional Spectrum of Perimenopause

The hormonal turbulence of perimenopause isn't just about hot flushes and periods. It's a full-blown **emotional storm** — and women are often caught in it without a life vest.

Here are some of the most common emotional and mental health symptoms:

- **Irritability and rage**: Often out of proportion and hard to control
- **Anxiety and panic attacks**: Even in women with no previous history
- **Sadness and crying spells**: Sometimes over a coffee ad… or nothing at all
- **Emotional detachment**: Feeling numb, disconnected from family or work
- **Overwhelm and burnout**: The feeling of drowning in tasks and emotions

Why does this happen?
Fluctuating oestrogen directly affects neurotransmitters like **serotonin, dopamine, and GABA,** which regulate mood, energy, and calmness. When oestrogen dips unpredictably, so does our emotional stability.

What the Research Says About Coping Tools

Let's explore the **evidence-based tools** that actually help calm the emotional chaos of perimenopause:

1. Mindfulness & Meditation

Mindfulness is the practice of being fully present —
observing your thoughts and feelings without judgment.

- **Harvard study (2018)**: Women who practiced
  mindfulness had **significantly lower anxiety and
  improved mood** scores during perimenopause.
- **JAMA Internal Medicine (2014)**: Mindfulness-
  based stress reduction (MBSR) was linked to
  improved sleep, mood, and reduced hot flushes
  in midlife women.

Try this simple 4-7-8 Breathing Technique:

1. Inhale through your nose for 4 seconds
2. Hold your breath for 7 seconds
3. Exhale slowly through your mouth for 8 seconds
4. Repeat 4–6 times

This activates your **parasympathetic nervous system**,
signalling your body to relax.

Proven Meditation Techniques for Perimenopause Relief

Meditation isn't just "woo-woo wellness." It's
neuroscience. Regular practice can help regulate your
**nervous system, reduce cortisol, boost serotonin and
dopamine**, and even **reshape your brain**.

Here are **five research-backed meditation techniques** that
are particularly helpful during perimenopause:

- ## Mindfulness Meditation (MBSR)

What it is:
You focus on the present moment — your breath, bodily sensations, sounds — and gently return your attention every time your mind wanders.

How to practice:

- Sit quietly for 5–20 minutes.
- Focus on your breathing.
- When thoughts come, acknowledge them and gently return to your breath.

Why it works:
Harvard studies show that MBSR reduces anxiety, hot flushes, and even insomnia during perimenopause. It increases grey matter in brain regions linked to memory and emotional regulation.

- ## Body Scan Meditation

What it is:
Progressive relaxation and awareness of bodily sensations from head to toe.

How to practice:

- Lie or sit comfortably.
- Close your eyes.
- Slowly scan each body part — from your scalp to your toes — noticing tension and releasing it.

Why it works:
A 2020 study in Psychosomatic Medicine found body scans improved sleep and reduced physical tension in women with midlife stress.

- ## Loving-Kindness Meditation (Metta)

What it is:
You silently send well wishes to yourself and others: "May I be safe. May I be well. May I be at peace."

How to practice:

- Begin with yourself.
- Then extend these wishes to a loved one, a neutral person, someone you're struggling with, and finally the world.

Why it works:
Journal of Women's Health (2019) reported significant improvements in **self-compassion**, **emotional resilience**, and **reduced depressive symptoms** in menopausal women.

- ## Mantra Meditation

What it is:
You repeat a word or phrase — silently or aloud — to centre your mind.

How to practice:

- Choose a word like "peace," "calm," or the Sanskrit "so hum" (meaning "I am").

- Sit quietly and repeat it with your breath.

Why it works:
NCCIH clinical trials have shown that mantra meditation helps reduce **blood pressure**, **anxiety**, and **mental chatter** in midlife women.

▪ <u>Guided Meditation (Apps & Audio)</u>

What it is:
You follow an instructor's voice guiding you through imagery, relaxation, or affirmations.

Best for beginners or those with an overactive "monkey mind."

Recommended apps:

- **Insight Timer** (free with great menopause meditations)
- **Headspace**
- **Balance** (offers perimenopause programs)
- **Ten Percent Happier** (science-based)

Meditation and Hormones

Research shows meditation:

- **Lowers cortisol** (the stress hormone)
- **Stabilises mood swings** by enhancing serotonin pathways

- **Improves oestrogen balance** indirectly by improving adrenal function and reducing inflammation

Menopause Journal (2022) concluded that women who meditate 10+ minutes a day report **less brain fog**, **better sleep**, and **greater emotional clarity**.

Start Where You Are

You don't have to sit like a monk on a mountain. You can meditate in your bed, on your office chair, even during a hot flush in the car.

Start with 2–5 minutes. Set a timer. Be consistent. Progress, not perfection.

2. Journaling

Writing isn't just self-expression — it's therapy. Journaling helps you:

- Process emotions
- Identify patterns in symptoms and mood
- Release pent-up frustration in a healthy way

University of Rochester research found that journaling **reduces stress and improves clarity**, especially in women dealing with emotional overwhelm.

Try this prompt:

"Today I felt angry when... but beneath that anger, I was really feeling..."

3. Therapy and CBT (Cognitive Behavioural Therapy)

CBT is a well-studied approach to managing perimenopausal symptoms, especially emotional and cognitive ones.

📚 **The British Menopause Society** supports CBT for:

- Hot flushes and night sweats
- Anxiety and depression
- Sleep disturbances
- Emotional regulation

Even 4–6 sessions can lead to **significant improvement in quality of life**.

4. Community Support

You are not meant to go through this alone.

Support groups — online or in person — reduce isolation, normalise the experience, and offer practical advice from other women walking the same path.

Studies show that **peer connection** improves emotional resilience, self-esteem, and even adherence to treatment plans.

Tip: Start a WhatsApp group, join a Facebook community, or simply gather two friends for a monthly "real talk" session.

The Healing Power of Hobbies

Crocheting a unicorn may seem silly. But in that meditative repetition, I found space. Stillness. Healing. Crafts, art, gardening, puzzles — anything that requires gentle focus and brings joy — can **regulate mood and rewire your brain**. This is called **occupational mindfulness**.

This was my blog post back in 2021:

"Since the on and off lock down since last year march due to COVID, the kids have not gone to school almost a year and their classes are being conducted online. What that means is they are in the house 24hours! I as a parent had to come up with all sorts of activities to keep them occupied and also to keep their mental health in check. It is not easy for kids to be staring at the laptop/computer for 8 hours, and not having any physical interaction with their friends, it can do a number on them. I had to learn the hard way that my plans can sometimes backfire on me when most of the time they insist on including me in those activities lol!

So my daughter and I started to crochet in April of 2021. The hooks and yarns are pretty affordable, and I would dare say cheap y'all. So we sat down and learned the basics, and it was nice having a partner and she picked it up faster than I did(nope that did not hurt my ego, at all!). We even tried knitting, and this I included my mother and sister who were living in another state. We used to meet up over zoom or facetime every Sundays and that was a great idea. But the knitting was not for me, so I stuck to crocheting.

I found while I crochet, I become focused, and you have to though or else you will miss some stitches. I found that by focusing, my crazy mind was getting quiet, almost like meditating, and I can't meditate to save my life! Little did I know, this crochet business was going to be my saviour at the most chaotic time of my life!

Did you know that research have been conducted to study the benefits of crocheting in conditions such as anxiety and dementia?

A study which was conducted by Michelle Borst Polino found several benefits of crocheting and knitting such as:

1. Knitting and crocheting relieves depression

2. Crafting reduces anxiety

3. Projects build self-esteem

4. Crafting may reduce or postpone dementia

5. Knit and crochet through insomnia

6. Relaxation reduces irritability and restlessness

7. Crafting as prayer

8. Yarncrafting builds community

9. Crafting helps with grief processing

10. stress busting benefits of yarncrafting

Isn't that just fantastic? Who would have known right? So for all the negatives that came out of this COVID infection and lockdown...this was definitely a plus point! So join me on my journey on crocheting and how it made a huge difference in my life.

I love this quote:
"Every single second is an opportunity to change your life, because in any moment you can change the way you feel" Rhonda Bryne

Looking back, I was 40 years old in 2020, and I was clearly going through perimenopause and I did what I could to cope for not just my sake but for the sake of my children. They needed me, but more that I realised, I needed them. They were my support, and they helped me through all that.

"Sometimes clarity doesn't come from fixing things. It comes from stepping back and being still."

Summary — How to Ride the Emotional Waves

Tool	Why It Works
Mindfulness / Meditation	Reduces cortisol, stabilises mood, improves sleep
4-7-8 breathing	Activates parasympathetic nervous system for calm
Journaling	Externalises emotion, identifies triggers, promotes self-reflection
CBT / Therapy	Offers tools to reframe negative thoughts and improve resilience
Hobbies (crochet, art)	Induces flow state, supports emotional regulation
Support groups / Friends	Validates experience, reduces shame, builds community

"Why did I cry over a coffee ad?" Because your hormones are playing DJ with your emotions. And you, my dear, are dancing through it like a warrior."

Chapter 5: Taking Control of Your Body

Feeling Strong: Reclaiming Strength in Perimenopause

I've always been petite.

At my heaviest — 69 kg — I was pregnant with my son. But even then, it wasn't just fat. It was water retention. I remember the nurse telling me they couldn't even feel my spine. That's how swollen I was.

I lost 10 kgs within a week after delivery, and that told me something — my body wasn't about overeating or indulgence. It was something deeper. Hormonal. Metabolic.

Even though I've never been obese, I know what it feels like to look in the mirror and not recognise yourself. As someone with a small frame, even a few extra kilos made me look rounder, softer — and not in a way that felt good. **The belly fat, the bloating, the flabby arms** — it all crept in slowly, even though I was doing "the right things."

I started playing tennis at 35. I hit the gym. I did yoga, which helped but I also learned that I had tight hips and I am not that flexible, which is really frustrating. I tried swimming when I could. I was also picky with food, I have always been a picky eater since young. And yet... I still had a FUPA(Fat Upper Pubic Area) that refused to budge and arms that felt jiggly no matter how many reps I did. And it didn't help when people who I meet say "eh gained some weight ah?" (a typical Asian way of saying how are you, I haven't seen you in a while). My son once told me I have body image issues. Maybe he's right, but can you blame me though? But let's be honest — **what woman doesn't wrestle with her body at some point, especially in her 40s?**

What's Really Happening to Your Body in Perimenopause?

It's not just calories in, calories out. Here's what the science says:

Hormonal Shift	Impact on Body
• ↓ Oestrogen	Increases fat storage, especially in the abdomen
• ↓ Progesterone	Causes water retention and bloating
• ↑ Cortisol (from stress)	Encourages central fat and insulin resistance
• ↓ Muscle mass (sarcopenia)	Reduces metabolism, increases body fat percentage

So no, it's not in your head. That stubborn belly? That bloating? That softening? **It's biology.**

What Finally Worked for Me: Tennis, Pilates & Intermittent Fasting...and Yoga

Pilates: The Game Changer

When I started Pilates, when I was 45, I wasn't expecting a miracle — but what I got was power. Real, physical power.

I felt **toned, leaner and stronger**. It wasn't about weight loss anymore — it was about **body confidence**.

Research says:
A 2021 meta-analysis in *Menopause* found that **Pilates significantly improved core strength, posture, flexibility, and body image** in women aged 40–60. It also reduced lower back pain and improved pelvic floor tone — something many perimenopausal women struggle with.

Benefits of Pilates for Perimenopausal Women:

- Increases lean muscle mass
- Improves pelvic floor and posture
- Enhances flexibility and joint stability
- Boosts confidence and reduces anxiety

Tip: Start with reformer or mat-based classes 2–3x per week. You'll feel results in 4–6 weeks.

Intermittent Fasting: Control Without Starvation

I started **intermittent fasting (IF)** because I needed structure. I wasn't bingeing. I wasn't dieting. But I needed a **reset**. And IF gave me that.

It wasn't just about shrinking the number on the scale — it was about **rebalancing my body and mood**.

Science behind IF in women 40+: A 2022 study in *Obesity Reviews* found that **time-restricted eating (16:8 method)** in perimenopausal women led to:

- Reduction in waist circumference

- Better insulin sensitivity
- Lower inflammation markers
- Improved energy and sleep quality

Tips for Intermittent Fasting:

- **Start with 14:10** (14 hours fast, 10-hour eating window), then move to 16:8
- Break your fast with **protein + fibre** (e.g. eggs + avocado + greens)
- Stay hydrated with water, herbal teas, or black coffee during fasts
- Avoid sugar binges in your eating window — **quality matters**

🚫 **Warning:** IF may not be suitable if you have a history of eating disorders or adrenal fatigue. Always listen to your body.

Yoga: Flexibility, Flow, and Finding My Centre

I committed to yoga for more than six months. My goal? To improve my flexibility. Simple things — like sitting cross-legged on the floor or touching my toes — felt like Olympic events. My hips were tight, my hamstrings even tighter, and I started to wonder: is this just me, or is something anatomically off?

The more I practiced, the more I realised — this wasn't just about stiffness. My pelvis seemed tilted, and my posture felt… off. And it turns out, I wasn't imagining it.

What the Research Says:
A 2020 review in *Menopause* found that yoga significantly improved flexibility, balance, and musculoskeletal function in perimenopausal and postmenopausal women. But it also noted something deeper: yoga helped correct **pelvic misalignment** and **postural asymmetries**, which can become more noticeable as muscle tone and oestrogen levels decline.

Women in perimenopause often develop **tight hip flexors, glute weakness, and anterior pelvic tilt** — all of which can contribute to:

- Lower back pain
- Pelvic floor dysfunction
- Decreased mobility
- Inability to fully forward bend or sit comfortably on the floor

Benefits of Yoga for Perimenopausal Women:

- Improves pelvic alignment and postural balance
- Enhances flexibility, especially in hips and hamstrings
- Reduces joint pain and muscle stiffness
- Supports emotional regulation and sleep quality
- Lowers cortisol (stress hormone), easing anxiety and mood swings
- May reduce vasomotor symptoms like hot flushes

Tip: Start with gentle hatha or restorative yoga. Focus on poses like *pigeon, child's pose, cat-cow,* and *forward fold.* Consistency is key — even 15 minutes a day adds up.

Personal insight: Yoga didn't turn me into a human pretzel, far from it. But it gave me the grace to meet my body where it is. And slowly, gently, my flexibility improved but not that much. I think I need to do it more often to get to where I want, in terms of flexibilty. Persistence is the key.

The Secret Supplement: Creatine for Women Over 40

Yes — **creatine**. Not just for gym bros.

A 2021 review in *Nutrients* confirmed that **creatine helps perimenopausal women:**

- Preserve and build muscle mass
- Improve cognitive function (yes, memory!)
- Increase bone density
- Support performance and recovery from exercise

How to take it:

- 3–5g per day of **creatine monohydrate**
- Take it **with food or after your workout**
- **No loading phase required**
- Safe and well-tolerated — no, it doesn't "bulk you up"

Think of creatine as your **muscle-preserving, brain-boosting secret weapon**.

Other Nutrition Tweaks That Help

Change	Why It Matters

Change	Why It Matters
Increase protein to 1.2–1.5g/kg	Supports muscle, reduces hunger, stabilises blood sugar
Cut back on processed carbs	Prevents insulin spikes and inflammation
Focus on magnesium & omega-3s	Reduce PMS, anxiety, and bloating
Eat more fermented foods	Supports gut health → reduces bloating, boosts mood

Summary: You Can Reclaim Your Body

What Worked for Me	Why It Helps
Pilates	Builds strength, improves tone, boosts confidence
Intermittent Fasting (IF)	Reduces central fat, resets metabolism, boosts energy
Creatine	Supports muscle, brain, and bone health after 40
Balanced eating	Protein + fibre + healthy fats = hormonal harmony

"Your body is not misbehaving — it's changing. But with the right tools, you can meet it where it is and thrive."

Chapter 6: Sex, Intimacy, and Libido — The Untold Struggles

When the Bedroom Goes Quiet — and So Do We

Of all the chapters, I found this one the most difficult to write. It is not easy to talk about intimate topics, but I think this needs to be discussed.

I met my husband when I was just 20 — two medical students, in a foreign country, and an intense crash into love. It was real, exciting, unpredictable — as young love often is. He was my dark knight on a white horse!

The funny thing is, growing up I always said "I never want to get married! I never want to have children!" Well the moral of this story is "never say never!".

Back to the plot twist, we eventually got married after 7 years and we built a life with our two beautiful children. And somewhere in the mess and miracle of parenthood, exams, long working house, and stress — **something between us started to fade**.

It wasn't just the arguments, the silence, or the disconnection. It was the feeling of **being alone while not actually being alone.** I didn't know what I wanted. I didn't know how to ask for what I needed. And I certainly didn't feel understood and supported. What made everything worse was that I kept isolating myself. I did not know what else to do.

Then, as I turned 40, another silence crept in — **my libido left me.** I'm not being poetic — it was abrupt, cruel, and complete. She divorced me when I was 43. Wait who? I am talking about my selfish libido who just left and didn't leave a note.

"Is This Normal?" — The Grief of a Lost Sex Drive

Let's be honest — no one prepares you for this. Not your mother. Not school. Not your GP.

One day you feel mildly "not in the mood." Then it becomes weeks. Then months. Then you find yourself actively avoiding touch — not because you don't love your partner/husband, but because your **body no longer responds**. And you don't know why. It's difficult to talk about this because the conversation ultimately turns to "is it me?" How can you make someone understand what is going on with you when you don't understand it yourself?

What made it worse? **Seeing women on social media** raving about their husbands. Weekend getaways. Flirty captions. Reels where they're all over their man. And here I am, ashamed, envious, confused. What is wrong with me?

When Sex Actually Hurts

There were times I *forced* myself to be intimate, hoping the act would awaken something in me. Instead, it left me **in pain — literally tearing pain.** How can an act of love leave me crying? And I don't mean happy crying! And the worse part, I do this silently so I don't upset my husband.

No man wants to see his wife in tears after sex unless it's happy tears. I didn't have happy tears, sex was causing me so much pain it was unbearable.

Back in my late 30s, I started experiencing **post-coital bleeding**(bleeding after sex) **and pain**. I did my CST (cervical screening test), and it came back normal. So I went to my gynaecologist— expecting understanding, reassurance… maybe an explanation.

She laughed and said "Well everything looks normal, maybe your husband is too rough," and then said, "Just kidding." I was mortified!

But it wasn't funny. It was humiliating.

She never asked if I had vaginal dryness. Never explored hormonal causes. Never took my pain seriously.
And here's the truth that I later learned in my own women's health training in Australia:
Vaginal dryness is real.
Painful sex is real.
And no one should be laughed at for experiencing it.

The Hormone Nobody Talks About: SHBG

For some reason I decided to check my hormones and noticed my **SHBG (sex hormone-binding globulin)** was high. I didn't know what it meant back then. But here's what I've come to understand:

SHBG is a protein made by the liver. SHBG binds to sex hormones like **testosterone and oestrogen**, making them inactive. Think of it like putting your hormones in handcuffs.

In perimenopause:
- SHBG levels may **increase** (especially if you're on the pill, have liver conditions, or high oestrogen exposure).
- High SHBG means **less free testosterone** — and that's a problem, because **free testosterone** is critical for **libido, energy, and sexual responsiveness**.

So if you feel "numb," flat, and uninterested in sex — it may not be psychological. It may be **biochemical**.

The Intimacy We Don't Talk About

Losing libido isn't just about missing sex — it's about **missing connection**.
The cuddles that don't lead to pressure.
The kisses that don't lead to guilt.
The feeling of being *wanted*, but not being able to *want back*.

This can lead to:

- Resentment
- Distance
- Miscommunication
- Self-blame

"It's not you being cold. It's your hormones going silent."

What You Can Do — Treatments & Options

Medical Options

Concern	Treatment
Vaginal dryness / pain	Local vaginal oestrogen (cream, pessary, ring) — safe, even long term
Loss of libido	Consider testosterone therapy (topical), if low and symptomatic
Low oestrogen / SHBG high	Evaluate hormone profile with GP; may benefit from systemic HRT
Painful penetration	Use lubricants (water- or silicone-based), vaginal dilators if needed

Australian Menopause Society supports vaginal oestrogen as safe and effective for genitourinary syndrome of menopause (GSM), even in women with a history of hormone-sensitive cancers (with oncologist input).

Natural & Lifestyle Options

- **Coconut oil or hyaluronic acid vaginal moisturisers** (non-hormonal, daily use)
- **Mindful sex / Sensate focus exercises** — reconnect with non-penetrative touch
- **Pelvic floor physio** — improves circulation, lubrication, and tension-related pain
- **Sleep, nutrition, stress reduction** — all impact sexual health and hormone regulation

Rekindling Intimacy — Slowly, Gently, Honestly

- Talk to your partner — even if it's hard. Explain what's happening and what you need.
- Schedule "non-sexual intimacy" — cuddling, massages, touch without expectations.
- Explore connection-building outside the bedroom — laughter, quality time, affirmations.
- Seek couples therapy if needed — it's a strength, not a weakness.

"Rebuilding intimacy isn't about going back to how it was — it's about meeting each other where you are now."

Summary: Sex May Change — But It's Not Over

Issue	You're Not Alone — and Here's What Helps
Low libido	Check SHBG, testosterone, explore testosterone therapy
Vaginal pain or dryness	Local oestrogen, lubricants, vaginal moisturisers
Feeling disconnected	Reframe intimacy, communicate, rebuild emotional closeness
Shame or confusion	Educate yourself — your body is not broken, it's changing

"If no one has told you this yet: you are not less of a woman because you don't want sex. Your worth is not measured by your libido. But you deserve answers, and you deserve care."

Chapter 7: Lost in the Fog — My Story and the Science Behind Brain Fog

"I just read this yesterday—why can't I remember it?"

If someone had asked me in my early 30s whether brain fog was real, I would've laughed it off. But now? I've lived it.

I started my GP fellowship when I was 35. I had the roadmap planned perfectly: study hard, pass each step, and become a specialist by the time I turned 40. The program was designed to take 4.5 years.

It took me 7 years.

Seven long years.

Every morning, I woke up at 5 AM to study before the world in my house stirred. I was a physician, a practice owner, a wife, a mother, and a homemaker — roles I wore all at once, with very little room to breathe.

And yet, despite all the hours I poured into my books, I kept forgetting things. I'd read something one day and it would vanish from my memory the next. Every exam failure triggered an avalanche of self-loathing:

"Why am I so stupid?"
"Why can't I retain anything?"
"Why did I start this so late in life?"

I felt like my brain had betrayed me. I thought I was burnt out. I thought maybe I just wasn't cut out for this. What I didn't know then — what I know now — is that I was in the middle of **perimenopause**, and the brain fog I was experiencing was very, very real.

What Is Brain Fog?

"Brain fog" isn't a clinical diagnosis, but that doesn't make it any less valid. For many women, it feels like:

- Walking into a room and forgetting why
- Struggling to find the right words mid-sentence
- Losing focus during simple tasks
- Forgetting appointments or daily routines
- Feeling "slower" or mentally cloudy

You're not lazy. You're not losing your mind. **You're perimenopausal.**

Studies show that up to **60% of women in perimenopause** report cognitive difficulties, especially around memory and attention span.

In my 40s, I'd be mid-conversation, and the word I needed would just… disappear. Like it had been abducted by my own brain. I'd look at the person I was talking to, frozen, waiting for the right word to arrive.

Sometimes I'd laugh it off with:

"I'm losing my mind! Must be getting older."

It helped to joke about it — but honestly? It was shaking my self-esteem. I even started to understand why my mother would rattle off every name under the sun before landing on mine.

I thought it was hilarious when I was younger.

Now? Not so funny.

Why Does Brain Fog Happen in Perimenopause?

As oestrogen fluctuates and declines, it disrupts how the brain functions:

Neurotransmitter Changes

Oestrogen supports **serotonin**, **dopamine**, and **acetylcholine** — all critical for mood, memory, and focus. Without it, mental sharpness dulls.

Brain Fuel Disruption

Oestrogen helps neurons use **glucose** efficiently. When levels drop, your brain literally struggles to access energy — like trying to run a car on fumes.

Sleep Disruption

Night sweats, insomnia, and even undiagnosed **sleep apnoea** interrupt memory consolidation and reduce mental clarity.

Mood Disorders

Anxiety and depression — more common during perimenopause — impair cognitive function even further.

A 2013 Harvard study (Epperson et al., *Journal of Neuroscience*) confirmed that perimenopausal women had reduced brain activation during memory tasks compared to premenopausal women.

The Real-Life Impact

Brain fog might seem like a minor nuisance from the outside, but it can **dismantle your confidence and disrupt your life**.

In Work:

- Making small errors
- Forgetting patient names or protocols
- Feeling like an imposter

In Relationships:

- Zoning out during conversations
- Forgetting important dates or routines
- Withdrawing out of fear or embarrassment

In Motherhood:

- Missing school events
- Forgetting homework tasks
- Feeling disconnected or inadequate

For high-achieving women — especially in medicine, education, or caregiving — it can be devastating.

How to Treat and Manage Brain Fog

The good news? There are **evidence-based strategies** that can help.

Medical Treatments

Hormone Replacement Therapy (HRT):

- Endorsed by the *Australian Menopause Society* for improving cognitive symptoms
- Works best when started **under age 60** or within **10 years of menopause**
- May support memory and neural efficiency
- *Note: HRT is not approved for dementia prevention*

SSRIs/SNRIs:

- If anxiety or depression are contributing, antidepressants can help regulate mood and improve cognitive clarity

Lifestyle & Cognitive Strategies

- **Prioritise sleep**: Address insomnia and evaluate for OSA
- **Exercise**: Aerobic activity increases hippocampal volume (brain's memory centre)
- **Mindfulness & Meditation**: Proven to reduce cortisol and improve attention
- **CBT**: For addressing shame, anxiety, and mental overwhelm

Nutritional and Natural Supports

- **Omega-3 fatty acids**: May improve memory and reduce brain inflammation
- **Vitamin B12 & D**: Deficiencies can mimic brain fog
- **Ashwagandha**: An adaptogen shown in studies to improve stress response and resilience
- **Limit alcohol**: It impairs sleep and memory

Practical Tools for Daily Life

- Use **phone reminders**, **planners**, or **voice notes**
- Break big tasks into smaller, manageable steps
- Use humour — like I did — to deflect tension when words escape you
- Most importantly: **be kind to yourself**
  This is biology, not a flaw in your character

When to Seek Medical Review

While brain fog is common, speak to your doctor if you experience:

- Progressive memory loss
- Getting lost in familiar places
- Difficulty with daily tasks
- Severe mood changes or disorientation

Possible medical mimics:

- Early-onset dementia

- B12 deficiency
- Thyroid dysfunction
- Major depression

Quick Reference Table: Clearing the Fog

Action	Why It Helps
Start HRT (if eligible)	Stabilises oestrogen, improves neural communication
Prioritise sleep	Restores memory consolidation processes
Exercise regularly	Improves blood flow and brain function
Use CBT or therapy	Manages anxiety, shame, emotional load
Supplement B12, D, Omega-3	Restores nutrients essential for cognition
Try adaptogens (Ashwagandha)	May reduce cortisol and improve focus under stress
Laugh when you forget	Diffuses tension, connects you to others
Be compassionate with self	Because this isn't your fault — it's your hormones

Final Thought

If you feel like your brain is broken — it's not.
It's just **reprogramming itself**.

This fog doesn't last forever. But even while you're in it,
you can find tools that work for *you*.

Because knowledge isn't just power — **it's permission**.

Permission to rest.
Permission to treat.
Permission to stop blaming yourself and start supporting
yourself.

Chapter 8: Fatigue, Freezing, and Falling Apart — When Perimenopause Mimics Everything Else

I was 35 when I first felt like something was deeply off. My skin started drying out. I was *so* tired — not just tired, but bone-tired, soul-tired. I was constipated all the time, and please don't get me started on the hair loss. It wasn't just a few extra strands in the shower — it was literal handfuls. I chalked it up to stress from work and the endless hours of studying. After all, I was running a clinic, raising children, managing a household, and training for my fellowship. Of course I was exhausted… right?

But no matter how much I slept, how clean I ate, or how many supplements I threw down — I wasn't coping.

Eventually, I checked my thyroid and iron levels. The results came back: **subclinical hypothyroidism and iron deficiency anaemia.** I remember staring at the results and thinking, "Well, that explains a lot." I started on **thyroxine** just to feel like I could function. It helped *a little*, but the iron tablets were a nightmare — they made my constipation even worse. Some days, I'd bleed from straining on the toilet. Now I had a whole new problem on top of my existing ones.

After four years on thyroxine, the palpitations became unbearable. I had to stop. I now check my levels regularly, and to my surprise — **everything has normalised.** It wasn't until much later that I realised what had been happening all along.

It was **perimenopause.**

Perimenopause, Thyroid Function, and Iron Deficiency — What Does the Research Say?

Perimenopause and Thyroid Dysfunction

1. The Symptom Overlap Is Real

What's often dismissed as "just hormones" might actually be your thyroid waving a red flag. The **symptom overlap** is uncanny:

- Fatigue
- Weight gain
- Brain fog
- Mood swings
- Cold intolerance
- Constipation
- Menstrual changes
- Hair thinning

This overlap means thyroid disorders are often **misdiagnosed or overlooked** in perimenopausal women.

2. Hormone Interaction: Oestrogen and the Thyroid

Oestrogen affects **thyroid-binding globulin (TBG)** — the protein that transports thyroid hormones. During perimenopause:

- Fluctuating oestrogen alters TBG levels.
- This can affect **free T3 and T4**, the active thyroid hormones.
- As a result, some women appear "normal" on labs, but feel anything *but* normal.

Evidence spotlight: A 2021 review in *Climacteric* reported that **TSH levels tend to rise with age** and thyroid dysfunction is often under-recognised in perimenopausal women due to its symptom overlap.

3. Autoimmunity and Age

Perimenopause also coincides with a spike in **autoimmune thyroid conditions**, including:

- **Hashimoto's thyroiditis**
- **Graves' disease**

Declining oestrogen is known to alter immune regulation, triggering or worsening autoimmune tendencies.

Perimenopause and Iron Deficiency
1. The Bleeding Nobody Talks About

Perimenopause often brings:

- **Anovulatory cycles** → unopposed oestrogen → **heavy or prolonged periods**
- **Shorter or irregular cycles**
- **Clotting, flooding, and surprise bleeds**

This chronic blood loss leads to **iron deficiency**, often without anaemia — just *low ferritin*, which still affects:

- Energy
- Mood
- Cognition
- Hair growth
- Thyroid function

Research: A 2020 study in *AJOG* found that **25% of perimenopausal women with fatigue had undiagnosed iron deficiency**, even when haemoglobin was normal.

2. Iron Is Essential for Brain and Thyroid Health

- Iron is a **cofactor for thyroid hormone production** (especially T4 → T3 conversion).
- It's also vital for **dopamine and serotonin** — the very chemicals that regulate mood and focus.

So if your **iron is low**, your **thyroid struggles**, your **brain fog worsens**, and your **mental health tanks**.

What Does This Mean in Practice?

Symptom	Possible Cause	Tests to Consider
Heavy periods	Perimenopause, anovulatory cycles	FBC, ferritin, pelvic ultrasound

Symptom	Possible Cause	Tests to Consider
Fatigue + brain fog	Iron deficiency, thyroid dysfunction	Ferritin, TSH, free T4, B12, Vitamin D
Anxiety or depression	Hormonal shifts, low iron or thyroid	Iron studies, thyroid panel, mental health screen

Women with fatigue, cognitive changes, or menstrual irregularities in their 30s or 40s deserve **more than "it's just hormones."** They deserve a **workup.**

Summary — What You Need to Know

Finding	Backed by
Thyroid dysfunction can mimic perimenopausal symptoms	Australian Menopause Society, Endocrine Society
Autoimmunity risk rises with age	Immunology and endocrinology research
Perimenopausal bleeding leads to chronic iron loss	AJOG, Women's Health journals
Iron deficiency worsens brain fog, mood, and thyroid function	Nutritional and psychiatric studies

Finding	Backed by
Screening is essential: ferritin, TSH, free T4, B12, and FBC	Standard practice guidelines

Before you blame your brain — check your iron. Before you blame your hormones — check your thyroid.
And before you blame yourself — know this: It's not just stress. It's your biology trying to talk to you.

Chapter 9: The Gallbladder Surprise — When Perimenopause Hits Below the Belt

A Personal Tale of Unexpected Pain

Let me tell you another story — we all love stories, right?

Back in my medical school days, I was no stranger to gastritis. Surviving on coffee, skipping meals, and enduring high stress made antacids my go-to remedy. Fast forward to my late 30s and early 40s, during my GP Fellowship, the familiar gnawing pain intensified. Antacids no longer sufficed, leading me to proton pump inhibitors (PPIs).

By the time I turned 42, amidst relocating to Australia, the abdominal pain became sharper and more frequent. A food intolerance test revealed allergies to yeast, almonds, and potatoes — goodbye pizza, French fries, and whiskey. Despite dietary adjustments, the pain persisted.

One day, while exercising, a sudden central chest pain struck. Fearing a heart attack, I rushed to the hospital. The culprit? A 2.7 cm gallstone.

I was stunned. I didn't fit the typical profile: over 40, overweight, or with a family history of gallstones. Yet, here I was, facing surgery. My surgeon warned, "If we don't remove it, it could corrode the gallbladder wall and turn cancerous." The 'C' word was enough to convince me.

Post-surgery(I had a keyhole surgery) my surgeon comes into my room to check up on me. He said "the stone was huge amu, I had a hard time extracting it. But strange thing is, it was a pigmented gallstone. Do you have any history of a bleeding disorder?" He hands the container with the stone to me, and I am staring at this stone with shock!

Wait... a Pigmented Stone?

My gallstone wasn't just large — it was **2.7 cm** and **pigmented**. That detail didn't mean much to me at the time, but later, curiosity got the better of me. I had to know: *What exactly is a pigmented stone?* And why did I have it? And no I did not have any history of a bleeding disorder.

By the way, there are more than one type of gallstone — and they each tell a different story about your body.

The Three Main Types of Gallstones

1. Cholesterol Stones

- **Description:** Made mostly of hardened cholesterol
- **Appearance:** Yellow-green, smooth
- **Causes & Risk Factors:**
  - Obesity
  - High-fat diet
  - Oestrogen dominance (e.g. HRT, pregnancy, perimenopause)
  - Diabetes
- **Frequency:** ~80% of cases (most common type)

2. Pigment Stones (Black)

- **Description:** Made of bilirubin and calcium salts
- **Appearance:** Small, black, brittle
- **Causes & Risk Factors:**

- o Chronic haemolysis (e.g. sickle cell anaemia)
  - o Liver disease
  - o Ageing
- **Frequency:** Less common

3. Pigment Stones (Brown)

- **Description:** Mixture of cholesterol and calcium salts
- **Appearance:** Soft, brown, greasy
- **Causes & Risk Factors:**
  - o Biliary infections
  - o Parasitic infestations (more common in Asia)
- **Frequency:** Rare

Mixed Stones

- **Description:** Combination of cholesterol and pigment components
- **Appearance:** Variable
- **Causes & Risk Factors:** Combination of the above (cholesterol and pigment stone) risk factors
- **Frequency:** Variable

What Are Pigmented Stones?

There are **two types** of pigmented stones:

1. **Black Pigmented Stones**
   - Form in **sterile bile**
   - Often associated with **chronic haemolytic diseases, cirrhosis**, and **aging**
2. **Brown Pigmented Stones**
   - Form in **infected bile ducts**
   - More common in **East Asian populations** and in settings with biliary infections or parasites

You probably guessed it — **pigmented stones are less common** than cholesterol stones, but **not rare**, especially in Asian women. Studies show an increased incidence of pigmented stones in women during **perimenopause and menopause**, possibly due to:

- Changes in **bile composition**
- **Stagnant bile flow** due to declining oestrogen
- Metabolic shifts, **increased oxidative stress**, and mild liver dysfunction during the perimenopausal transition

Research Insight

A study published in *Hepatology International* (2022) showed that:

"Women aged 40–55, especially those in perimenopause with fluctuating oestrogen and progesterone, showed higher incidence of pigmented gallstones in Asian cohorts, regardless of BMI or cholesterol levels."

This supports what many of us in midlife medicine are starting to see — **you don't need to be overweight or**

unhealthy to get gallstones during this transition. The hormonal chaos of perimenopause can be enough.

The Hidden Link: Perimenopause and Gallstones

So, why did I develop a gallstone despite lacking common risk factors? Emerging research suggests that perimenopause itself may be a contributing factor.

Oestrogen's Role
During perimenopause, fluctuating estrogen levels can disrupt bile composition, increasing cholesterol saturation and reducing bile acid secretion. This imbalance promotes gallstone formation. Additionally, estrogen can impair gallbladder motility, leading to bile stasis — a known risk factor for gallstones.

Progesterone's Impact
Elevated progesterone levels, common in perimenopause, may further slow gallbladder emptying, compounding the risk.

Hormone Replacement Therapy (HRT)
While HRT alleviates menopausal symptoms, studies indicate that oral estrogen therapy increases gallstone risk. Transdermal applications (patches or gels) may pose a lower risk, but caution is advised.

Prevention and Management Strategies

Understanding the connection between perimenopause and gallstones empowers us to take proactive steps:

1. *Dietary Adjustments*

- **Increase Fiber Intake**: A diet rich in fruits, vegetables, and whole grains supports healthy digestion.
- **Healthy Fats**: Incorporate sources like avocados and nuts to promote bile flow.
- **Limit Refined Carbs and Sugars**: Reducing these can decrease cholesterol levels in bile.

2. *Regular Physical Activity*

Engage in consistent exercise to maintain a healthy weight and support overall digestive health.

3. *Hydration*

Adequate water intake ensures bile remains fluid, reducing the risk of stone formation.

4. *Monitor Hormone Therapy*

If considering HRT, discuss the risks and benefits with your healthcare provider, and explore transdermal options to potentially lower gallstone risk.

5. *Regular Medical Check-ups*

Routine screenings can detect early signs of gallbladder issues, allowing for timely intervention.

What Can We Do?

Knowing the type of stone helps tailor future management and prevention strategies:

- **Cholesterol stones** may benefit from dietary changes and weight management.
- **Pigmented stones** often signal an underlying bile flow or liver-related issue — so liver health, hormonal balance, and **regular follow-up** is essential.

Final Thoughts

I never thought I'd need my gallbladder story to help other women — but here we are.

If you're a perimenopausal woman with unexplained gut pain, don't dismiss it as "just gastritis" or stress. Listen to your body. Ask questions. Get imaging.

A pigmented gallstone may not be typical — but then again, **nothing about perimenopause ever is**.

Chapter 10: The Symptoms No One Warns You About

The Not-So-Obvious Signs of Perimenopause (That Are Absolutely Real)

Let's face it — when we think about menopause, the media shows us a woman fanning herself, maybe snapping at her husband, and then moving on with life. But the truth is far more nuanced.

Not all symptoms of perimenopause come with a flashing neon sign that says "HORMONES." Some sneak up quietly. Others are misunderstood, misdiagnosed, or dismissed entirely — even by healthcare professionals. So let's talk about them.

Real Struggles We Don't Talk About

1. *Recurrent UTIs (and the agony that comes with them)*

By the time women hit their 40s, many start noticing more frequent urinary tract infections — even if they had never experienced them before. The culprit? Genitourinary Syndrome of Menopause (GSM).

As oestrogen declines, the tissues lining the bladder, urethra, and vaginal canal become thinner, drier, and more fragile. This creates a perfect storm for bacterial overgrowth and irritation.

What helps:

- Local vaginal oestrogen: pessaries, creams, or vaginal rings (safe and effective)
- Non-hormonal moisturisers: look for hyaluronic acid-based or pH-balanced options
- Hydration: increase water intake
- Avoid soaps or douches: especially those with fragrance
- Cranberry extract & probiotics: limited evidence, but generally safe
- Always get a urine culture before antibiotics. Not all "UTIs" are infections — some are due to irritation.

Did you know? Vaginal oestrogen is safe for many breast cancer survivors — speak to your specialist.

2.Allergies, Itchy Ears, and Oestrogen's Sneaky Role

Think it's odd that your allergies are worse? Or that your ears itch more than usual? You're not imagining it.

Oestrogen is deeply involved in the immune response and histamine regulation. As levels fluctuate during perimenopause, many women experience:

- Worsening seasonal allergies
- New sensitivities to foods or chemicals
- Dry or itchy ears
- Post-nasal drip or sinus issues

What helps:

- Non-sedating antihistamines
- Nasal steroid sprays or moisturising ear drops

- Hormonal balance: through HRT or natural supports
- Check your environment: new home? new pet? Hormonal sensitivity can uncover hidden triggers.

3.Foot Pain & Joint Stiffness

That morning heel pain? The sudden achiness in your knees? How about the severe joint pains 1 week before you periods? Yep — perimenopause might be the villain.

Oestrogen has anti-inflammatory effects on joints. As levels drop:

- Collagen declines
- Tendons stiffen
- Plantar fasciitis and joint pain become common

What helps:

- Stretching and yoga
- Resistance training
- Consider a bone density scan if fractures or chronic pain occur

4.Dizziness and Heart Palpitations

I always get dizzy and always blamed it on my low blood pressure and low iron. What worried me was the palpitations and chest pain. I would be lying down at night, and my heart would be racing. I don't suffer from anxiety but the palpitations were making me anxious. I decided to have a stress test done because I have a strong family history of heart disease and guess what, all normal. This is important to note because you need to check yourself out thoroughly before blaming it on one thing. Don't just assume it's perimenopause, check your heart out!

Back to perimenopause symptoms, some women report feeling dizzy, lightheaded, or like their heart is racing. This isn't always anxiety — it can be due to:

- Fluctuating oestrogen's effect on blood vessels
- Drops in iron or B12
- Perimenopausal POTS(Postural orthostatic tachycardia Syndrome)-like symptoms

What helps:

- Get tested: ECG, iron studies, B12, thyroid
- Mindfulness to manage vasovagal symptoms
- Salt/electrolyte balance if fainting or low BP is an issue

5.Vaginal Flatulence (Queefing): The Embarrassment No One Talks About

Let's get real: you're in yoga class, mid-downward dog, and suddenly... a sound escapes from *down there*. It even happens when you stand up after sitting for some time, or walking, or laughing!!! It's not gas. It's not a fart. But it sounds like one.

Welcome to **vaginal flatulence**, also known as **queefing** — the audible release of trapped air from the vaginal canal. It's not harmful. It's not dirty. It's not even rare. But it can be **embarrassing as hell**.

Why does it happen, especially now? As we age and go through perimenopause, the following changes can make queefing more noticeable:

- **Loss of vaginal tone:** Declining oestrogen can cause the pelvic floor muscles and vaginal walls to weaken and become less elastic.
- **Vaginal dryness and atrophy:** The walls become thinner and more prone to allowing air pockets.
- **Position changes:** Yoga, sex, squatting, or certain forms of exercise can force air into the vaginal canal, which escapes when you move again.
- **Post-birth anatomy:** Women who have delivered vaginally may experience more frequent queefing due to stretching of the vaginal canal or pelvic floor dysfunction.

What does the research say? While vaginal flatulence isn't often discussed in clinical trials, pelvic floor physiotherapists and women's health researchers link queefing with:

- Pelvic floor muscle dysfunction or weakness (Rosenbaum, 2007)
- Vaginal laxity associated with hormonal changes (Pastore et al., 2010)
- Decreased oestrogen levels and resulting atrophy (NAMS, 2022)

How to manage or prevent queefing:

- **Pelvic floor physiotherapy (PFPT):** Kegels alone are not enough — targeted pelvic floor work with a trained therapist can improve tone and control.
- **Vaginal oestrogen therapy:** Helps restore vaginal wall integrity and elasticity.

- **Pessary devices:** In some cases, they help with support and tone.
- **Body positioning:** Modify exercise postures or sexual positions to reduce the chance of air trapping.
- **Don't hold shame:** It's a mechanical response, not a reflection of hygiene or health.

Bottom line? You didn't "fail to clench." Your pelvic floor may just need support. Well at least now we know why it happens and we also know that all is not lost. There are things we can do to make it better.

Chapter 11: Why Managing Perimenopause Matters — More Than Just Hot Flushes

Most people think of perimenopause as nothing more than a nuisance. A few hot flushes. Some mood swings. A bit of weight gain. It'll pass, right?

But what many women—and even some healthcare providers—don't realise is that **untreated or unrecognised perimenopausal symptoms can lead to serious, chronic health conditions** that impact not only quality of life but long-term mortality.

This chapter will explore the **medical consequences of unmanaged perimenopause**, backed by research and clinical guidelines.

Hormone Chaos = Systemic Effects

During perimenopause, the body undergoes **fluctuating and eventually declining oestrogen levels**. Oestrogen plays a role in nearly every major body system, so when it begins to fall, the effects ripple out widely.

These hormonal changes can lead to:

- **Sleep disturbances**
- **Weight gain**, especially visceral (belly) fat
- **Mood instability**
- **Reduced insulin sensitivity**
- **Dysregulated cortisol and stress response**

These symptoms, when left unmanaged, are not "just a part of getting older"—they can lead to significant **health risks**.

1. Weight Gain and Metabolic Syndrome

Multiple studies show that **perimenopausal women experience an increase in central adiposity**—fat stored around the abdomen. This isn't just cosmetic.

According to the *Study of Women's Health Across the Nation (SWAN)*, oestrogen decline leads to a **redistribution of body fat**, increasing visceral fat and decreasing lean muscle mass.

Consequences of untreated weight gain:

- Insulin resistance and **type 2 diabetes**
- Elevated LDL cholesterol and **atherosclerosis**
- Increased risk of **ischaemic heart disease** (the number one killer of women in Australia)

Australian Institute of Health and Welfare (AIHW) data supports that cardiovascular disease becomes more prominent in women after midlife, often coinciding with the hormonal shift of menopause.

2. Sleep Disorders and Obstructive Sleep Apnoea (OSA)

Many perimenopausal women report **difficulty falling or staying asleep**. This is often dismissed as "normal," but the impact can be dangerous.

Oestrogen and progesterone influence:

- Respiratory drive

- Upper airway muscle tone
- REM sleep stability

Declines in these hormones can lead to or **worsen undiagnosed OSA**, especially in women with:

- Weight gain
- Snoring or night-time gasping
- Excessive daytime fatigue

Untreated OSA increases the risk of:

- **Hypertension**
- **Stroke**
- **Heart disease**
- **Cognitive decline**

In women, OSA is often underdiagnosed because it presents with fatigue and mood symptoms rather than loud snoring.

3. Depression, Anxiety, and Mental Health

The **perimenopausal transition is a vulnerable time for developing mood disorders**.

Studies (Freeman et al., JAMA Psychiatry, 2014) confirm that perimenopausal women have:

- **2 to 4 times higher risk** of developing major depressive episodes
- Increased **anxiety, irritability, and emotional dysregulation**

The risk is higher in women with:

- Past history of depression

- Severe PMS or PMDD(Premenstrual Dysmorphic Disorder)
- Poor social support
- Sleep disturbances

Untreated, this may progress to:

- Severe depression
- Relationship breakdown
- Suicidality
- Loss of employment and self-worth

4. Bone Loss and Osteoporosis

Oestrogen is crucial for bone density maintenance. During perimenopause and menopause:

- Women lose **2–5% of bone mass per year**
- Osteoporosis risk **doubles post-menopause** without intervention

This leads to:

- Fragility fractures
- Long-term disability
- Increased morbidity and hospitalisation in older women

According to Osteoporosis Australia, one in two women over 60 will suffer an osteoporotic fracture.

The Fracture That Made Me Pause

When I was 43, I was training hard for a women's tennis tournament — possibly the fittest I'd been since delivering my daughter 13 years ago. Three days after my birthday, I was running backward to return a lob. I didn't notice a stray ball on the court.

I stepped on it, lost balance, and fell hard on my left side. I landed on my bum and outstretched wrist. I heard the crack before I felt the pain.

A trip to the hospital confirmed it — an **undisplaced fracture of my left wrist**.

I'd never fractured anything in my life. And though the fall seemed innocent, something about it didn't sit right. Was this just bad luck… or **early osteoporosis**?

I'm now investigating my bone health. My **vitamin D has always been low**, and that fall felt like more than a fluke.

According to Australian guidelines, **any woman over 50 who experiences a minimal trauma fracture** should be screened for **osteoporosis** with a DEXA scan — even if they feel "young" or healthy.

It made me realise: **bone loss isn't something that creeps in after 70**. It starts earlier — often silently — and unless we catch it early, the first sign might be a fracture. I obviously did not fit into the age group of developing osteoporosis, or was I?

What the Guidelines Say: Osteoporosis and Fractures in Midlife Women

Any fracture after age 50 should raise a red flag for possible osteoporosis, especially if it results from a low-trauma event (like slipping or falling from standing height). Even if the fracture is **non-hip or non-vertebral**, it still significantly increases the risk of future fractures.

Clinical Practice Guideline Recommendations:

1. **Automatic Bone Density Assessment (DEXA)**
   - Women ≥50 years old who experience a **minimal trauma fracture** should undergo **bone mineral density testing** (DEXA scan).
   - A prior fracture is considered a **clinical risk factor** regardless of T-score.
   - Vitamin D, calcium, and fracture risk assessment tools (e.g. **FRAX** or **Garvan**) should also be used.
2. **Start Treatment If Osteoporosis Is Diagnosed**
   - First-line treatment: **Bisphosphonates** (e.g., alendronate, risedronate)
   - Alternatives: **Denosumab** (especially in women with GI intolerance), **raloxifene**, or **HRT** (if indicated for other menopausal symptoms and no contraindications)
3. **Recurrent Fracture Prevention**
   - Early management after first fracture reduces risk of future fractures by **30–70%**.
   - Fracture liaison services (FLS) are encouraged to systematically follow up post-fracture patients.

What to Do After a Fracture in Perimenopausal/Postmenopausal Women

Step	Action	Purpose
1.	DEXA scan	Assess bone density
2.	Serum calcium, phosphate, ALP, Vitamin D, TSH, renal & liver function	Rule out secondary causes
3.	Start calcium (1000–1300mg/day) & vitamin D if low	Support bone metabolism
4.	Consider pharmacologic therapy if T-score ≤ -2.5 or if fragility fracture present	Prevent further fractures
5.	Lifestyle: weight-bearing/resistance exercise, Smoking cessation, alcohol moderation	Bone health and fall prevention

AMS Insight: *HRT is considered protective against osteoporosis **before age 60 or within 10 years of menopause** and can be a first-line option for prevention in women with menopausal symptoms and increased fracture risk.*

Why Early Intervention Matters

By recognising and managing perimenopause **early and holistically**, we can:

Symptom	Management	Long-term Prevention
Weight gain	Diet, exercise, HRT, metformin (if insulin resistance)	Prevent T2DM, CVD
Sleep disturbance	CBT-I, HRT, melatonin, OSA assessment	Prevent fatigue, mood disorders, stroke
Mood changes	HRT, therapy, SSRIs if indicated	Reduce depression, improve QoL
Bone loss	HRT, calcium, vitamin D, resistance training	Prevent fractures, preserve mobility
Vasomotor symptoms	HRT or non-hormonal therapies	Improve sleep, mood, work function

This Is a Turning Point, Not the End

Too many women are told, *"It's just your hormones, wait it out."* But research tells us this approach is **clinically negligent**.

Addressing perimenopause:

- **Protects your brain, heart, and bones**
- **Improves your relationships and work performance**
- **Empowers you to take charge of your health in midlife and beyond**

"Perimenopause is a biological warning light—not a weakness. When we acknowledge it, we can treat it. When we treat it, we can prevent disease." — *Australian Menopause Society*

Chapter 12: Alternative and Complementary Therapies

From Ashwagandha to Acupuncture — Navigating Natural Support with Wisdom

After all that trauma and drama I finally moved to Australia end of 2023. I came with more than just two teenage kids and a shipping container of belongings — I carried the full weight of **exhaustion, anxiety, hormonal chaos**, and the worry of having to handle it all without a support system.

The most daunting part? **Housework.** I'd never done it all by myself — no helper, no extended family, no cushion. I was already tired. How would I manage?

And then, I discovered **Chemist Warehouse** — a paradise for every supplement-curious and skin care fanatic woman like me. Somewhere between the magnesium and the multivitamins, I picked up a bottle of **ashwagandha**, a herb I remembered reading about in Ayurvedic medicine. My mindset was: "Why not try something?"

Ashwagandha: My Daily Ritual

Since **September 2023**, I've taken ashwagandha every morning with water — right before my coffee. It didn't feel like a magic bullet, but it **lifted the fog**. After a few weeks, I noticed:

- I could manage my clinic duties *and* return home to cook, clean, and parent without collapsing.

- I didn't need to crawl into bed by 8pm with zero energy.
- I still had tired days, yes — but not the soul-draining, wipe-you-out exhaustion that had become my norm.

It helped me function. It helped me *cope*. And that, at the time, was more than enough.

What the Research Says About Ashwagandha

Ashwagandha (*Withania somnifera*) is classified as an **adaptogen** — a plant that helps the body adapt to stress and restore balance.

Evidence-based insights:

- A **2019 double-blind placebo-controlled study** found that 600 mg/day of ashwagandha extract **lowered cortisol** and improved **stress resilience**.
- Studies suggest it **enhances mitochondrial energy production**, which may reduce fatigue and brain fog.
- Some evidence also supports improvements in **mood**, **sleep**, and **mental clarity** in midlife women.

Caution: Ashwagandha should be taken under medical supervision if you have thyroid conditions, autoimmune diseases, or are on sedatives.

According to the **Australian Menopause Society**, there is *emerging but limited* evidence for herbal adaptogens in perimenopausal women. The Society does not officially endorse any herbal therapy but acknowledges that some women may find subjective benefit.

For Period Mayhem and Hormonal Storms

Another challenge that hit me hard after 40? **My periods turned into horror movies.** Gushing on Day 1 and 2, cramps that curled me in bed, **depression**, **joint pain**, **acne**, and **hot flushes** that came a week before my period even started.

So I reached for **Black Cohosh** — another herbal remedy known for managing hormonal symptoms.

After **3 months** of taking it, I was stunned:

- My periods became manageable
- No more crawling into bed at 8pm
- No hot flushes, no joint pain

I felt like I had a part of my life back — although my **emotional motivation** and **joy at work** hadn't quite returned. Still, this was progress I could feel.

What the Research Says About Black Cohosh

Black Cohosh (*Actaea racemosa*) is one of the most studied herbal therapies for menopausal symptoms.

Evidence summary (AMS & NAMS):

- May relieve **vasomotor symptoms** like hot flushes and night sweats in some women.
- Its exact mechanism is unclear but **does not appear to have oestrogenic effects**.
- Effects may be seen after 8–12 weeks of consistent use.

However:

- Not effective for everyone
- Some women report **gastrointestinal side effects or headaches**
- There is **insufficient long-term safety data**, especially in women with hormone-sensitive cancers

AMS position: *Black Cohosh may offer symptom relief for some women, but **should not be considered a substitute** for medical treatment when HRT is clearly indicated.*

Other Natural and Lifestyle Options — What's Worth Trying?

Therapy	Evidence-Based Effect	AMS View
Yoga	Reduces hot flushes, anxiety, improves flexibility and sleep	Supported as part of lifestyle management
Meditation	Helps with anxiety, mood swings, emotional regulation	Helpful adjunct, especially for mood-related symptoms
Acupuncture	May reduce hot flushes and sleep	May provide benefit for some women; safe when supervised

Therapy	Evidence-Based Effect	AMS View
	disturbances (mixed evidence)	
CBT (Cognitive Therapy)	Strong evidence for managing anxiety, insomnia, and hot flushes	Recommended, especially for women not eligible for HRT
Hypnosis	Some evidence for hot flush relief	Emerging therapy — more research needed

Supplements That Might Help — and Those That Might Not

Supplement	Evidence & Role
• **Magnesium**	May help with anxiety, sleep, and muscle tension
• **Vitamin D & Calcium**	Crucial for bone health during and after menopause
• **Omega-3s (Fish Oil)**	May reduce inflammation, support mood and cognition

Supplement	Evidence & Role
• **Phytoestrogens (Soy, Red Clover)**	Mild symptom relief for hot flushes in some; inconsistent results
• **Evening Primrose Oil**	Minimal evidence for menopause symptom relief; not generally recommended

✖ *Avoid "menopause detox teas" or miracle cure powders — these often lack scientific backing and may interfere with medications.*

Final Thoughts — Natural Doesn't Mean Passive

Choosing natural or complementary therapies isn't about doing less — it's about doing what's **aligned with your body, your values, and your journey.**
For me, that meant starting with supplements like ashwagandha and Black Cohosh.
For others, it might be CBT, acupuncture, or yoga.
For some, it's HRT.
And for most — it's **a little bit of everything.**

Summary: What Works — and How to Choose Wisely

Treatment	Best For	Evidence Level
Ashwagandha	Stress, energy, mood	Moderate (emerging)
Black Cohosh	Hot flushes, heavy periods, aches	Moderate (short term only)
Yoga & Meditation	Mood, sleep, flexibility	Strong
CBT	Mood, sleep, vasomotor symptoms	Strong
Acupuncture	Hot flushes, sleep (variable)	Mixed
Soy / Red Clover	Mild symptom relief (some women)	Mixed

"Just because it's natural doesn't mean it's weak. And just because it's medical doesn't mean it's wrong. Find what works for you — science and self can coexist."

Chapter 13: To HRT or Not to HRT? That Is the Question

Weighing Hormone Therapy with Heart, Head, and Hormones

I never thought I would consider Hormone Replacement Therapy (HRT).

I had the same questions my patients ask me:
"Is it safe?"
"Won't it cause cancer?"
"Aren't I too young?"
"Shouldn't I just tough it out?"

And for a while, I did try to tough it out. The hot flushes were annoying but manageable. The mood swings made me think I was losing my mind. The fatigue made me question my career. And the libido? Well, she'd packed her bags and ghosted me.

As a GP, I knew HRT was an option. But as a woman in my 40s, I felt conflicted. So I started researching harder — for myself and my patients. What I discovered was surprising:
HRT has changed. The science has evolved. And for many women, it's life-changing.

But First — Let's Clear Something Up

Before we go any further, let's make one thing **very clear**:
HRT is not contraception.

If you are in perimenopause and still menstruating — even irregularly — **you can still get pregnant**, even if you're on HRT.

This surprises a lot of women.

Why? Because HRT and the **combined oral contraceptive pill (COCP)** both contain oestrogen and progestogen. But they're designed for completely different purposes:

Feature	Combined Pill (COCP)	HRT (Combined or Oestrogen-only)
Primary Purpose	Contraception	Menopause symptom relief
Hormone Dose	**High** (suppresses ovulation)	**Low** (replaces deficient levels)
Cycle Control	Yes	Not consistently
Prevents Ovulation	✔ Yes	✘ No
Pregnancy Prevention	✔ Yes	✘ No
Available As	Tablet	Tablet, patch, gel, pessary, ring

Bottom line:
If you are under 51, still getting periods, and not confirmed menopausal (12 months without a period), **you still need contraception.**

So if you're in perimenopause, experiencing symptoms, and need both **contraceptive protection and symptom relief**, here's what we usually recommend:

What's Best for a Woman in Perimenopause With Regular Cycles?

For a woman in her 40s with an intact uterus, still cycling (even irregularly), and experiencing perimenopausal symptoms:

Option 1: Combined Oral Contraceptive Pill (COCP)

- Higher hormone dose = contraception + symptom control
- Regulates bleeding, reduces hot flushes and mood swings
- Not suitable for women who smoke, have migraine with aura, or clotting risks

Option 2: Progestogen IUD (e.g. Mirena) + Oestrogen (patch/gel)

- Mirena provides endometrial protection and contraception
- Add low-dose oestrogen for symptom relief
- Excellent choice for heavy bleeding + contraception + HRT bridge

Option 3: Progestogen-only pill + Oestrogen patch/gel

- Useful if COCP is contraindicated
- May not provide regular bleeding control

Once you're 12 months period-free (natural menopause), you can then **transition to standard HRT** doses and formulations without worrying about contraception.

What Exactly Is HRT?

HRT — or Menopausal Hormone Therapy (MHT) — involves replacing oestrogen (and sometimes progestogen and testosterone) to relieve menopausal symptoms and support long-term health.

The Australian Menopause Society supports HRT as the most effective treatment for:

- Vasomotor symptoms (hot flushes, night sweats)
- Genitourinary symptoms (dryness, painful sex)
- Mood instability (in some cases)
- Sleep disturbance

And when started at the right time, HRT may also help reduce:

- Osteoporosis risk
- Cardiovascular disease (if initiated within 10 years of menopause)

When Is HRT Not the Right Choice?

HRT is generally not recommended in women with:

- Undiagnosed vaginal bleeding
- Active or recent breast cancer
- Known clotting disorders or recent DVT(deep vein thrombosis)/PE(pulmonary embolism)
- Untreated endometrial hyperplasia
- Significant liver disease

Use caution or specialist input in women with:

- Migraine with aura
- Strong family history of hormone-sensitive cancer
- Endometriosis
- Controlled hypertension

Matching HRT to Your Needs

Symptom	HRT Strategy
Hot flushes, night sweats	Systemic HRT (patch, gel, oral)
Vaginal dryness, painful sex	Local oestrogen (cream, pessary, ring)
Low libido (postmenopausal)	Add transdermal testosterone (specialist guided)

Symptom	HRT Strategy
Still has uterus	Combined HRT (oestrogen + progestogen)
No uterus	Oestrogen-only HRT
Early menopause (<45)	Strongly recommended until at least age 51

Safer options: Transdermal oestrogen + micronised progesterone = lower clot and breast cancer risk.

Why Progesterone Matters (If You Have a Uterus)

One thing that **must** be clear:

If you have an intact uterus and you're using systemic oestrogen, you must also take a progestogen. Always.

Progesterone **protects the endometrial lining** from unopposed oestrogen, which would otherwise increase the risk of **endometrial hyperplasia and cancer**.

- Micronised progesterone (body-identical) has the **lowest risk profile**
- Skipping it or "forgetting to refill" is **never safe**
- Vaginal oestrogen *alone* does not require progestogen — but systemic HRT does

Possible Side Effects of HRT — Know What to Watch For

Symptom	May Indicate	Action
Breast tenderness, bloating	Oestrogen dose may be too high	Review with GP
Breakthrough bleeding	Needs evaluation (especially after menopause)	Pelvic USG
Mood changes, insomnia	Progestogen side effect	Consider switching type/route
Leg swelling or calf pain	DVT warning	Urgent review
Headaches	May need alternative HRT formulation	Discuss with GP

My Personal Take

For me, HRT wasn't about "giving in" — it was about taking back control.

I needed energy. I needed clarity. I needed sleep. And I needed to feel like myself again — not a frazzled, foggy, tearful shadow of who I used to be.

For my patients, I don't push HRT. But I do present it fairly, honestly, and compassionately — because every woman deserves the full picture.

If you're still cycling and still confused — that's normal. Let's just make sure your treatment plan matches your **real life**, your **symptoms**, and your **goals**.

How Hormone Replacement Therapy Works

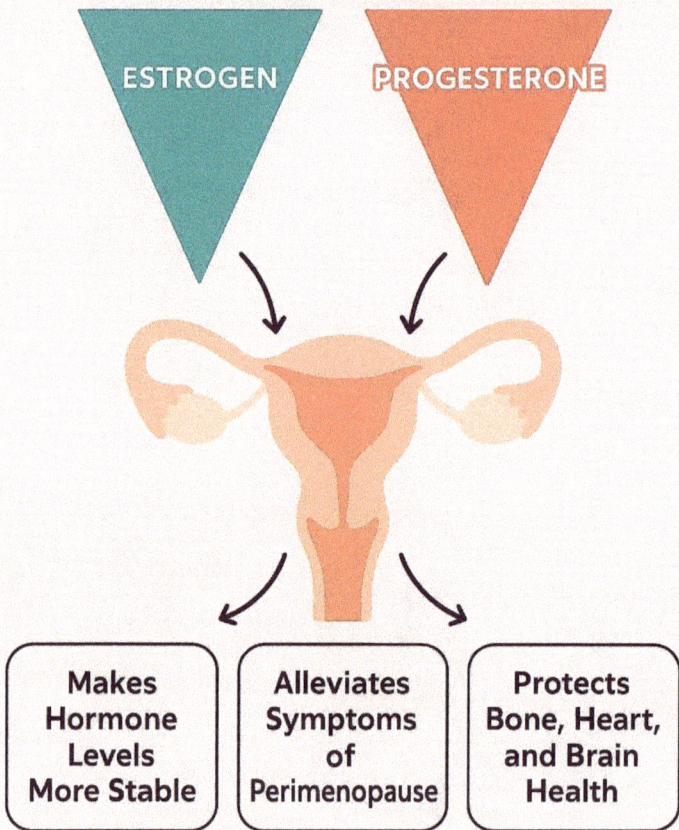

ESTROGEN

PROGESTERONE

Makes Hormone Levels More Stable

Alleviates Symptoms of Perimenopause

Protects Bone, Heart, and Brain Health

Chapter 14: The Preliminaries — What to Do Before Starting HRT

Empowerment Starts with Preparation

So, you're considering HRT. Maybe it's the insomnia. Maybe it's the hot flushes, the painful sex, or the constant irritability. Maybe you just want to feel **alive** again.

Before jumping into treatment, there's a checklist of important steps to ensure HRT is:

- **Safe**
- **Appropriate**
- **Tailored to you**

This is not about gatekeeping — it's about **doing it right**.

1. Comprehensive Medical History & Risk Assessment

Your GP should ask about:

- Age at symptom onset
- Menstrual cycle patterns (regular, erratic, stopped)
- Personal and family history (breast cancer, DVT, heart disease)
- Past use of contraception or hormone therapy
- Reproductive history: fibroids, endometriosis, hysterectomy
- Lifestyle factors: smoking, alcohol, BMI, physical activity

Tip: The AMS website offers risk calculators and decision aids to guide this.

2. Clinical Examination

- **Blood pressure**
- **Height and weight**
- **Breast exam** (and mammogram if due)
- **Pelvic exam** (if abnormal bleeding, pain, or dryness)

3. Blood Tests (If Indicated)

Routine hormone testing isn't necessary — but these may be considered:

Test	When to Order
FSH, LH,	Suspected early or premature
Oestradiol	Menopause (<45 yrs)
TSH, Iron, B12, Vit D	If fatigue, low mood, or poor concentration
Lipid profile, HbA1c	If metabolic risk factors are present
Testosterone, DHEAS	If evaluating low libido in postmenopausal women

4. Imaging & Screening — When It's Needed (Per RACGP & NCSP)

Alongside imaging, all women should be up to date with **age-appropriate national screening programs**:

Cervical Screening Test (CST)

- **Age:** 25–74 years
- **Frequency:** Every 5 years if HPV negative
- **Start:** 2 years after last Pap if transitioning
- **Delivery:** Clinician-collected or self-collection now available for eligible women
- *Important even after hysterectomy* if cervix is intact or there was a history of high-grade abnormality

Breast Screening (Mammogram)

- **Age:** 50–74 years (every 2 years) — **Free via BreastScreen Australia**
- **40–49 or >75:** Eligible on request

Bowel Cancer Screening

- **Age:** 50–74 years
- **Frequency:** Every 2 years (at-home FOBT kit)

Bone Density (DEXA Scan)

- Consider in women:
    - Over 50 with a **fragility fracture**
    - Early/premature menopause
    - Low BMI, corticosteroid use, smoking, or family history of osteoporosis

5. Mental Health & Lifestyle Review

Before starting HRT, ask:

- How's your sleep?
- Are you feeling anxious or down?
- Are you supported?
- Do you exercise, eat well, or drink alcohol regularly?

Sometimes addressing lifestyle first — or alongside HRT — can dramatically improve symptoms.

6. Clarify Your Goals & Preferences

Ask yourself:

- What symptoms are most affecting my life?
- Do I want hormonal or non-hormonal options?
- Am I seeking symptom relief, long-term health protection — or both?
- Do I have a uterus? (Hint: This decides whether you need **progesterone**)

Shared decision-making isn't just a phrase — it's a conversation that prioritises your values and needs.

Your Pre-HRT Checklist

Step	What to Review
Risk assessment	Medical, family, and lifestyle history
Physical exam	BP, BMI, breast, pelvic if indicated
Bloods	If clinically indicated
Imaging & Screening	Pelvic USG, mammogram, **cervical screening**, FOBT, DEXA scan if risk factors present
Mental health & lifestyle	Mood, sleep, diet, exercise, alcohol, support
Treatment preferences	Hormonal vs non-hormonal, delivery route, symptom goals

"HRT is not one-size-fits-all. It's your body, your choice — guided by evidence and empathy."

Conversations With My Patients

In my consultations with women over 30, I often ask them:

"Do you think you might be experiencing perimenopausal symptoms?"

Their responses are almost always the same:

"Maybe? I'm not sure…" "Am I in Menopause?"
"Wait — what exactly is that?"
"I didn't even know there was a name for what I'm feeling."

More often than not, these conversations end in tears. And I prepare for that moment — not because I expect sadness, but because I know what relief feels like when someone finally gets it.

That moment — when a woman feels truly seen and heard — is one of the reasons I love being a GP.

This isn't just about writing a script for HRT and sending someone on their way. It's about opening a door.

It's about offering knowledge, support, and most importantly — choices. Because when a woman understands what's happening with her body, and when she is given choices, she's empowered.

And that is where the journey back to herself truly begins.

Chapter 15: Building Your Personal Menopause Toolkit

Tools for Thriving — Not Just Surviving

Navigating perimenopause isn't a single moment — it's a journey. And every journey needs a map, a compass, and a backpack filled with essentials.

This chapter is about building your **toolkit** — the physical, mental, and emotional supports that make daily life feel a little more doable.

1. Journaling Prompts

- What is my body trying to tell me today?
- What was one thing that felt good this week?
- What do I need more of — and what can I release?
- How do I define strength right now?

Tip: Start with just 3 lines a day. Consistency beats perfection.

2. Symptom Tracker Ideas

Create a simple tracker with columns for:

- Sleep quality
- Mood (scale of 1–10)
- Period pattern
- Hot flushes
- Libido
- Exercise
- Nutrition

This helps you **notice patterns** and **guide treatment decisions**.

3. Self-Care Rituals

- A 10-minute walk at sunrise
- Evening chamomile tea and no screens after 9pm
- A weekly bath with Epsom salts and soft music
- Wearing lipstick or perfume — even on tired days

4. Books That Helped Me Feel Seen

- *The 5AM Club* — Robin Sharma
  Discipline that starts with self-respect
- *Think Like a Monk* — Jay Shetty
  Mental clarity and detachment
- *Happiness is Free* — Lester Levenson
  Letting go of suffering and embracing joy
- *How to Be Loved* — Humble the Poet
  Healing starts with self-acceptance

This isn't self-help fluff. These are anchors.

Chapter 16: Redefining Yourself in Your 40s and Beyond

Shifting Goals and Reclaiming Confidence

In my 30s, I was chasing timelines. I had mapped out my path to becoming a GP specialist before 40. Life had other plans — it took me seven years. I missed milestones. I missed sleep. I missed myself.

But somewhere along the way, I learned it wasn't about ticking boxes. It was about finding alignment.

In my 40s, alignment came in the form of purpose. I realised women's health wasn't just an interest — it was life changing. The silence around perimenopause was deafening. The lack of education and support was staggering. I saw a gap, and I stepped into it — for myself and for the women like me.

Perimenopause made my life very complicated, but it also peeled back the layers of who I thought I needed to be. And what I discovered underneath was someone more powerful than I imagined:

Resilient. Curious. Bold. Empathetic. Brave.

Reinvention didn't come in a neat package — it came through tears, questions, fatigue, and laughter. But it came.

And it brought with it a deep knowing:

This is who I am. This is what I'm here to do.

The Reinvention Begins With You

I've come to believe that everything happens for a reason. Every twist, every stumble, every hormonal meltdown — it all serves a purpose. And sometimes, that purpose takes a while to reveal itself.

Before moving to Australia, I often felt like I was floating in emotional limbo. Most of the women I connected with were either ten years younger — still figuring out life — or ten years older, already settled into their next chapter. The few friends my age were brilliant and busy, juggling demanding careers and families. No one really had the bandwidth to ask, "How are you?" And even if they did, I wouldn't have known where to begin.

I felt invisible — not just to others, but to myself.

Moving to Australia at 43 wasn't just a new job or a new location. It was a reset. A spiritual recalibration. I arrived burned out, emotionally frayed, and hormonally hijacked. But in the middle of all that chaos, I stumbled into something transformative: women's health.

As I stepped into this space as a GP, I began to recognise my own story in the women I treated. The hot flushes, the exhaustion, the loss of libido, the brain fog, the rage — it all made sense. For the first time, I had the language, the knowledge, and the tools to explain what had once felt like a personal failing.

And more importantly, I saw just how many women were quietly falling apart behind their well-curated lives. Just like I had.

This book? It's not just about me. It's about *us*. It's the honest conversation I wish someone had with me at 35 — when I thought I was going crazy, when my energy had evaporated, when intimacy became painful and my life felt like a hot mess.

I wrote this book to be the guide I desperately needed — and I hope it becomes that for you too.

Chapter 17: A Letter to My Younger Self... and My Daughter

What I Wish I Knew, and What I Hope You'll Remember

Dear Younger Me,

I know you're scared. You're trying to hold it all together — your studies, your career, your marriage, your children, your relationships. You've been taught to smile and keep going.

But let me tell you something: **being a woman is hard**. And no one gets to judge how you carry your pain.

There will be days when your body feels foreign, when your mind betrays you, and when your hormones rage like a storm. And the worst part? **No one will see it — because it's all invisible.**

But I promise: you're not weak. You're not crazy. You're just transitioning.

Don't isolate yourself, find your support, find your people, and ask for help, it's ok to ask for help.

You will make it. You will learn. You will come back to yourself — stronger, softer, wiser.

To My Daughter,

I see you — curious, radiant, hopeful. I never want you to be ashamed of your body or afraid of your biology.

Periods are not dirty.

Hormones are not shameful.

Mood swings don't make you unstable — they make you *human*.

I write this book for you. So you never have to walk blind like I did. So you'll be prepared, not scared. So you'll know what's happening when the fog sets in or the tears won't stop.

So you'll know that you're never alone.

"Knowledge is power. And knowing your body is the first revolution."

Acknowledgements

To every woman who has ever whispered, "What's happening to me?" — this book is for you.

I want to begin by thanking **my teenage children**, who were my anchors during a time when I was emotionally adrift. Your patience, humour, and quiet strength gave me reasons to keep showing up — even when I didn't feel like myself.

To my **patients** — the women who bravely shared their stories, tears, frustrations, and triumphs with me in the consult room — thank you. You reminded me that vulnerability is a strength, and that healing is often a shared journey.

To my **husband**, for the many versions of me you've stood beside — and to myself, for finally learning to stand tall for me.

Deepest appreciation to my mentors and colleagues in **women's health and general practice**, especially those in Australia who have helped shape my evidence-based, empathetic approach to menopause care.

To the **Australian Menopause Society**, thank you for your comprehensive, up-to-date clinical guidelines and resources. You've been the backbone of my professional understanding and a key compass in guiding this book.

And to **you**, dear reader — for choosing to understand your body, reclaim your voice, and seek answers that go beyond whispers and waiting. May this book be your mirror, your map, and your medicine.

References & Sources

The information presented in this book is grounded in peer-reviewed literature, clinical guidelines, and published evidence. Key references include:

Hormonal Changes, HRT, and Perimenopause

1. Australian Menopause Society. *AMS Information Sheets and Clinical Resources.* https://www.menopause.org.au
2. North American Menopause Society. *2022 Nonhormone Therapy Position Statement.*
3. The Study of Women's Health Across the Nation (SWAN). *NIH longitudinal data project on menopause and midlife aging.*
4. Davis, S. R., et al. (2015). *Global Consensus Statement on Menopausal Hormone Therapy.* Climacteric, 18(3), 231–235.

Complementary and Natural Therapies

5. Chandrasekhar, K. et al. (2019). *A prospective, randomized double-blind study of safety and efficacy of ashwagandha root extract in reducing stress and anxiety in adults.* Journal of Evidence-Based Complementary & Alternative Medicine.
6. Leach, M. J., & Moore, V. (2012). *Black cohosh for menopause symptoms: a systematic review of quality of trials and efficacy.* Maturitas, 72(4), 334–343.
7. Posadzki, P. et al. (2013). *Yoga for menopausal symptoms: A systematic review and meta-analysis.* Climacteric, 16(3), 336–345.

Brain Fog, Mood & Cognitive Function

8. Epperson, C. N., et al. (2013). *Effects of oestradiol on mood and cognition in perimenopausal and postmenopausal women: A randomized controlled trial.* Journal of Neuroscience, 33(48), 19071–19080.
9. Freeman, E. W., Sammel, M. D., Lin, H., et al. (2014). *Association of hormones and menopausal status with depressive symptoms in women.* JAMA Psychiatry, 71(1), 36–43.

Iron, Thyroid, and Metabolic Impacts

10. Climacteric Journal. (2021). *Thyroid dysfunction in midlife women: Clinical challenges and implications.*
11. The American Journal of Obstetrics and Gynecology. (2020). *Iron deficiency and fatigue in perimenopausal women.*

Lifestyle & Self-Development

- Robin Sharma. *The 5AM Club.*
- Jay Shetty. *Think Like a Monk.*
- Lester Levenson & Hale Dwonski. *Happiness Is Free.*
- Humble the Poet. *How to Be Loved.*
- Rhonda Byrne. *The secret*

Additional input and inspiration were derived from clinical experiences, women's health consultations, and ongoing CPD activities as part of professional general practice and menopause care in Australia.

www.ingramcontent.com/pod-product-compliance
Lightning Source LLC
Chambersburg PA
CBHW071234020426
42333CB00015B/1464